OSTEOTOMY SURGERY RECOVERY DIET

A Comprehensive Guide To Nourishing Your Body Through Nutrition For Rapid Recovering With Healing Recipes, Meal Plans, And Expert Tips For Long-Term Wellness

DR. ALLAN FREDA

Contents

Inside, readers will find a wealth of information tailored to support individuals newly diagnosed or undergoing osteotomy surgery.

From understanding the importance of nutrition in the healing process to practical strategies for implementing a recovery-focused diet, this book covers it all.

Key features include:

1.	Understanding the significance of nutrition in osteotomy surgery recovery: Learn about the specific dietary requirements essential for promoting healing and reducing the risk of complications post-surgery.

2.	Healing recipes: Explore a collection of delicious and nutritious recipes designed to support the body's healing process. From nutrient-rich smoothies to nourishing soups and wholesome meals, these recipes are tailored to meet the unique needs of individuals recovering from osteotomy surgery.

3.   Customized meal plans: Discover expertly crafted meal plans that take the guesswork out of meal preparation during the recovery period.

These plans are designed to provide optimal nutrition while accommodating any dietary restrictions or preferences.

4.   Expert tips for long-term wellness: Gain insights from healthcare professionals and nutrition experts on how to maintain a healthy lifestyle beyond the recovery phase.

Learn sustainable dietary habits and lifestyle practices that support overall wellness and prevent future complications.

With its comprehensive approach to nutrition and recovery, "Nourishing Recovery: A Guide to Osteotomy Surgery Diet" empowers individuals to take control of their health and well-being throughout the surgical journey and beyond. Whether you're preparing for surgery or navigating the post-operative phase, this book serves as a trusted companion for optimizing your recovery and achieving long-term vitality.

Disclaimer

The information in this book is for informational purposes only and should not replace professional medical advice, diagnosis, or treatment. Always consult your physician or a qualified health provider regarding any medical concerns. Do not disregard professional medical advice or delay seeking it based on information in this book.

The author does not endorse or have affiliations with any mentioned entities. References are for informational purposes only.

Consult your healthcare provider before making dietary or lifestyle changes, especially during recovery from surgery, as individual needs vary.

Results may vary, and the information provided is not guaranteed to produce specific outcomes.

By reading this book, you acknowledge and agree to consult your healthcare provider before implementing any information herein.

For further guidance, consult your healthcare provider or reputable medical websites for reliable information on surgery recovery diets.

CHAPTER 1
UNDERSTANDING OSTEOTOMY SURGERY AND RECOVERY

Osteotomy surgery is a procedure often recommended for individuals experiencing joint issues, particularly in the knees or hips.

This surgical intervention involves cutting and repositioning bones to improve alignment, alleviate pain, and enhance function. It's commonly used to treat conditions like osteoarthritis, hip dysplasia, and knee deformities.

The procedure aims to redistribute weight-bearing forces, reducing stress on damaged areas and promoting healthier joint mechanics. Recovery from osteotomy surgery can be challenging and typically involves a combination of physical therapy, medication, and lifestyle modifications.

One crucial aspect of this recovery process is nutrition, as it plays a significant role in supporting healing, reducing inflammation, and optimizing overall health.

Osteotomy surgery is a specialized orthopedic procedure designed to address structural abnormalities in bones, particularly in weight-bearing joints such as the knees and hips.

The term "osteotomy" is derived from two Greek words, "osteon" meaning bone, and "tomia" meaning to cut. During the surgery, the orthopedic surgeon carefully cuts and repositions the bone to correct alignment issues, relieve pressure on damaged cartilage, and improve joint function.

This realignment aims to redistribute forces across the joint, thereby reducing pain and delaying the progression of conditions like osteoarthritis.

The decision to undergo osteotomy surgery is often made after conservative treatments, such as medication, physical therapy, and lifestyle modifications, have proven ineffective in managing symptoms and preserving joint function. Candidates for this procedure typically experience persistent pain, limited mobility, and significant joint deformities that impact their quality of life. Common indications for osteotomy surgery include knee malalignment (varus or valgus deformity), hip dysplasia, and early-stage osteoarthritis.

The surgical technique employed may vary depending on the specific condition being treated and the patient's individual needs. For instance, in knee osteotomy, the surgeon may perform a high tibial osteotomy (HTO) or a distal femoral osteotomy (DFO) to correct varus or valgus alignment. In hip osteotomy, procedures such as a periacetabular osteotomy (PAO) or a femoral osteotomy may be performed to address acetabular dysplasia or femoroacetabular impingement (FAI).

Regardless of the type of osteotomy performed, the goal remains the same: to restore optimal joint mechanics, alleviate pain, and improve overall function. However, it's essential to recognize that osteotomy surgery is a major intervention that requires careful consideration of potential risks and benefits. Patients undergoing this procedure should be prepared for an extended recovery period and commit to following post-operative rehabilitation protocols to achieve the best possible outcomes.

Importance of Nutrition in Recovery

Nutrition plays a crucial role in the recovery process following osteotomy surgery. A well-balanced diet rich in essential nutrients is essential for supporting tissue healing, reducing inflammation, maintaining muscle mass, and promoting overall health and well-being. Proper nutrition can also help manage post-operative pain, enhance immune function, and facilitate the body's repair processes.

One of the primary nutritional goals during the recovery phase is to support tissue healing and repair. After osteotomy surgery, the body requires increased amounts of protein, vitamins, and minerals to rebuild damaged tissues, including bone, cartilage, and ligaments.

Protein, in particular, is essential for collagen synthesis, which is crucial for wound healing and tissue regeneration. Therefore, incorporating lean sources of protein such as chicken, fish, tofu, legumes, and dairy products into the diet is essential for promoting optimal recovery.

In addition to protein, vitamins and minerals also play critical roles in the healing process. Vitamin C, for example, is necessary for collagen formation and immune function, while vitamin D is essential for bone health and calcium absorption.

Minerals such as calcium, magnesium, and phosphorus are vital for bone formation and remodeling. Ensuring an adequate intake of these nutrients through a varied and balanced diet can help support the body's healing mechanisms and optimize recovery outcomes.

Another important aspect of nutrition during the recovery phase is the management of inflammation. Inflammation is a natural response to tissue injury and surgical trauma, but excessive or prolonged inflammation can impede the healing process and contribute to complications such as pain, swelling, and delayed wound healing.

Certain foods and nutrients have been shown to possess anti-inflammatory properties and may help mitigate post-operative inflammation.

These include omega-3 fatty acids found in fatty fish, flaxseeds, and walnuts, as well as antioxidants like vitamins A, E, and selenium found in fruits, vegetables, nuts, and seeds. Incorporating these anti-inflammatory foods into the diet can help reduce inflammation and promote faster recovery.

Maintaining a healthy body weight is also important for optimal recovery following osteotomy surgery.

Excess body weight can increase stress on the joints and impede healing while maintaining a healthy weight can help reduce strain on the surgical site and improve overall outcomes.

Therefore, adopting a balanced diet that provides appropriate caloric intake to support healing while preventing excessive weight gain is crucial for promoting long-term joint health and function.

In addition to supporting tissue healing and reducing inflammation, proper nutrition is essential for maintaining overall health and well-being during the recovery process.

Adequate hydration is critical for preventing dehydration and supporting cellular function, while a balanced intake of carbohydrates, fats, and fiber is necessary for sustained energy levels and digestive health.

Furthermore, certain dietary modifications may be necessary to address specific nutritional needs or restrictions following surgery, such as limiting sodium intake to reduce swelling or avoiding certain foods that may interfere with medication or exacerbate gastrointestinal issues.

Overall, nutrition plays a fundamental role in supporting recovery and optimizing outcomes following osteotomy surgery. By focusing on a well-balanced diet rich in essential nutrients, individuals can promote tissue healing, reduce inflammation, manage pain, and support long-term joint health and function. Consulting with a registered dietitian or healthcare professional can provide personalized guidance and support to help individuals develop a nutrition plan tailored to their specific needs and goals during the recovery process. With proper nutrition and diligent adherence to post-operative protocols, individuals can enhance their recovery experience and achieve optimal outcomes following osteotomy surgery.

CHAPTER 2
PREPARING YOUR KITCHEN FOR POST-SURGERY NUTRITION

Before delving into the specifics of a post-osteotomy surgery recovery diet, it's crucial to ensure that your kitchen is equipped with the necessary ingredients, tools, and equipment to facilitate a smooth transition to healthier eating habits. A well-prepared kitchen can significantly contribute to your recovery process, providing you with easy access to nutritious foods and simplifying meal preparation. Here's a comprehensive guide on how to prepare your kitchen for post-surgery nutrition.

Stocking your kitchen with essential ingredients is the first step towards maintaining a nutritious diet during your recovery period.

It's essential to focus on incorporating foods rich in vitamins, minerals, protein, and fiber to support your body's healing process and boost overall wellness. Here are some key ingredients to consider:

1.   Lean Protein Sources: Include lean protein sources such as chicken breast, turkey, fish, tofu, legumes, and eggs in your kitchen arsenal.

Protein is essential for tissue repair and muscle strength, both of which are crucial during the recovery phase.

2.   Whole Grains: Opt for whole grains like brown rice, quinoa, oats, and whole wheat bread and pasta. Whole grains provide sustained energy

and are rich in fiber, promoting digestive health and satiety.

3.   Fresh Fruits and Vegetables: Incorporate a variety of fresh fruits and vegetables into your diet to ensure you're getting a wide range of vitamins, minerals, and antioxidants.

Aim for colorful options like berries, leafy greens, citrus fruits, carrots, and bell peppers.

4.   Healthy Fats: Choose sources of healthy fats such as avocados, nuts, seeds, olive oil, and fatty fish like salmon and mackerel. Healthy fats are essential for brain health, inflammation reduction, and nutrient absorption.

5.   Low-Fat Dairy or Dairy Alternatives: If you consume dairy, opt for low-fat options like skim milk, Greek yogurt, and cottage cheese. Alternatively, choose dairy alternatives like almond milk, soy yogurt, and dairy-free cheese to accommodate dietary preferences or restrictions.

6.   Herbs, Spices, and Seasonings: Stock up on herbs, spices, and seasonings to add flavor to your meals without relying on excessive salt or sugar. Experiment with options like garlic, ginger, turmeric, cinnamon, and fresh herbs to enhance the taste of your dishes.

7.   Hydration Essentials: Don't forget to include hydration essentials like water, herbal teas, and electrolyte-rich beverages in your kitchen. Staying adequately hydrated is essential for overall health and can aid in the recovery process.

By ensuring that your kitchen is stocked with these essential ingredients, you'll have the foundation for creating nourishing meals that support your body's healing and promote long-term wellness.

Kitchen Tools and Equipment:

In addition to stocking essential ingredients, having the right kitchen tools and equipment can streamline meal preparation and make cooking more accessible, especially during the recovery period. Here are some key kitchen tools and equipment to consider:

1.   Blender or Food Processor: A high-quality blender or food processor can be incredibly versatile for preparing smoothies, soups, sauces, and purees.

These appliances make it easy to incorporate fruits, vegetables, and protein into your diet in easily digestible forms.

2.   Slow Cooker or Instant Pot: A slow cooker or Instant Pot can be a lifesaver for busy days or when you're not up to spending a lot of time in the kitchen. These appliances allow you to prepare nutritious meals with minimal effort, as you can simply add ingredients and let them cook slowly over time.

3.   Sharp Knives and Cutting Boards: Invest in sharp knives and durable cutting boards to make food preparation safer and more efficient. Having

the right tools can make chopping fruits, vegetables, and proteins much easier and reduce the risk of accidents in the kitchen.

4.   Nonstick Cookware: Nonstick cookware can make cooking and cleaning up a breeze, especially when you're dealing with limited mobility or energy during the recovery period.

Opt for high-quality nonstick pans and pots to minimize the need for excessive oil or butter when cooking.

5.   Meal Prep Containers: Investing in meal prep containers can help you portion out and store meals in advance, making it easier to stick to your nutritional goals and avoid relying on unhealthy convenience foods. Choose containers that are microwave-safe, dishwasher-safe, and stackable for easy storage.

6.   Kitchen Scale: A kitchen scale can be a valuable tool for portion control and ensuring accuracy when measuring ingredients, especially if

you're following specific dietary guidelines or recipes. It can also help you track your food intake and make adjustments as needed for optimal nutrition.

7.   Handheld Immersion Blender: A handheld immersion blender is a convenient tool for blending soups, sauces, and smoothies directly in the pot or container, eliminating the need to transfer hot liquids to a traditional blender. It's a handy gadget for creating smooth and creamy textures without much effort.

By equipping your kitchen with these essential tools and equipment, you'll be better prepared to tackle the challenges of meal preparation during the post-surgery recovery period. Having a well-stocked kitchen and the right tools at your disposal can make it easier to maintain a nutritious diet and support your body's healing process effectively.

CHAPTER 3
KEY NUTRIENTS FOR OSTEOTOMY SURGERY RECOVERY

Osteotomy surgery is a significant procedure aimed at correcting bone deformities or realigning bones to improve joint function. Following such surgery, a comprehensive approach to recovery, including proper nutrition, is crucial for optimal healing and rehabilitation. In this guide, we delve into the essential nutrients necessary for supporting recovery post-osteotomy surgery, focusing on protein, carbohydrates, and healthy fats.

Protein: Building Blocks for Healing

Protein stands as a cornerstone nutrient in the process of tissue repair and regeneration, making it vital for individuals recuperating from osteotomy surgery. Following surgery, the body's demand for protein escalates as it works to rebuild damaged tissues, including bones, muscles, and connective tissues. Adequate protein intake aids in the synthesis of new proteins, fostering the healing process and promoting muscle strength and function.

Lean sources of protein such as poultry, fish, lean cuts of meat, eggs, dairy products, legumes, and plant-based protein sources like tofu and tempeh are recommended for individuals recovering from osteotomy surgery. Incorporating protein-rich foods into each meal and snack throughout the day ensures a steady supply of amino acids, the building blocks of proteins, facilitating tissue repair and enhancing overall recovery.

Furthermore, it's essential to prioritize high-quality protein sources that offer essential amino acids necessary for optimal healing. Incorporating a variety of protein sources into the diet ensures a balanced intake of essential amino acids, supporting comprehensive recovery post-osteotomy surgery.

Carbohydrates: Energy for Recovery

Carbohydrates serve as the primary source of energy for the body, playing a vital role in fueling various physiological processes, including tissue repair and recovery. During the healing process following osteotomy surgery, the body's energy requirements may increase, necessitating an adequate intake of carbohydrates to support optimal recovery and rehabilitation.

Complex carbohydrates, such as whole grains, fruits, vegetables, and legumes, provide a sustained release of energy, helping to maintain stable blood sugar levels and support consistent energy levels throughout the day. These nutrient-dense carbohydrate sources also offer essential vitamins, minerals, and dietary fiber, contributing to overall health and well-being during the recovery period.

It's important to focus on consuming carbohydrates from whole, unprocessed sources to maximize nutrient intake and support optimal recovery post-osteotomy surgery.

Avoiding refined carbohydrates and sugary snacks helps prevent energy fluctuations and supports stable blood sugar levels, promoting sustained energy and optimal healing.

Healthy Fats: Supporting Overall Health

Healthy fats play a crucial role in supporting overall health and well-being, particularly during the recovery period following osteotomy surgery. Incorporating sources of healthy fats into the diet provides essential fatty acids, such as omega-3 and omega-6 fatty acids, which possess anti-inflammatory properties and contribute to the body's inflammatory response during the healing process.

Sources of healthy fats include fatty fish like salmon, mackerel, and sardines, as well as nuts, seeds, avocados, and olive oil. These foods offer a rich source of monounsaturated and polyunsaturated fats, which support cardiovascular health, reduce inflammation, and promote optimal healing and recovery post-osteotomy surgery.

Including a variety of healthy fats in the diet helps maintain proper cellular function, support hormone production, and enhance nutrient absorption, all of which are essential for comprehensive recovery and rehabilitation. Balancing the intake of healthy fats with other essential nutrients ensures a well-rounded approach to nutrition during the healing process following osteotomy surgery.

CHAPTER 4
CREATING BALANCED MEALS FOR RECOVERY

Undergoing osteotomy surgery can be a significant. event in an individual's life, often necessitating a comprehensive approach to recovery, including dietary considerations. A balanced diet plays a crucial role in supporting the healing process, promoting tissue repair, maintaining overall health, and enhancing the body's resilience. In this guide, we will delve into the importance of nutrition during osteotomy surgery recovery and provide practical insights into creating balanced meals for optimal healing and long-term wellness.

Creating Balanced Meals for Recovery

During the recovery period following osteotomy surgery, it's essential to prioritize nutrient-dense foods that provide the necessary vitamins, minerals, protein, and antioxidants to support tissue regeneration, reduce inflammation, and promote overall well-being. Crafting balanced meals ensures that your body receives the essential nutrients it needs to heal efficiently and effectively. A balanced meal typically consists of a combination of carbohydrates, protein, healthy fats, fiber, vitamins, and minerals, all of which play distinct roles in the healing process.

Breakfast serves as the foundation for your day, providing the energy and nutrients needed to kickstart your metabolism and fuel your activities. For individuals recovering from osteotomy surgery, a nourishing breakfast is particularly important as it replenishes energy stores and supports tissue repair.

Opt for whole-grain cereals or oats topped with fresh fruits, nuts, and seeds for a nutrient-rich start to your day. Alternatively, consider incorporating protein-rich foods such as eggs,

Greek yogurt, or tofu into your breakfast routine to support muscle recovery and promote satiety.

Smoothies made with leafy greens, fruits, and protein powder can also be a convenient and easily digestible option for those with reduced appetite or difficulty chewing.

Lunch Recipes for Sustained Nourishment

Lunchtime presents an opportunity to refuel your body midday and sustain energy levels throughout the afternoon. When planning your lunch meals during osteotomy surgery recovery, focus on incorporating a balance of lean proteins, complex carbohydrates, and healthy fats to support satiety and provide sustained nourishment.

Grilled chicken or fish paired with quinoa or brown rice and steamed vegetables make for a satisfying and nutrient-dense lunch option. Vegetarian alternatives such as lentil or chickpea salads with mixed greens, avocado, and a drizzle of olive oil offer a hearty dose of plant-based protein and essential nutrients. Additionally, homemade soups or stews loaded with vegetables, legumes, and lean proteins can provide comfort and warmth while promoting hydration and healing.

As the day winds down, dinner provides an opportunity to unwind and nourish your body with comforting and nutrient-rich meals.

When planning dinner recipes for osteotomy surgery recovery, prioritize foods that are easy to digest, rich in essential nutrients, and promote relaxation and restful sleep. Incorporating a variety of colorful vegetables, lean proteins, and whole grains into your dinner meals ensures that you receive a diverse array of nutrients to support healing and overall well-being. Consider preparing roasted vegetables with baked salmon or tofu and a side of quinoa or couscous for a simple yet nourishing dinner option. Alternatively, hearty vegetable-based stir-fries or pasta dishes with lean protein sources such as shrimp or turkey sausage offer a satisfying and flavorful way to end the day on a high note.

 prioritizing nutrition during osteotomy surgery recovery is essential for supporting the healing process, promoting overall well-being, and laying the foundation for long-term health and wellness. By focusing on creating balanced meals that are rich in essential nutrients, individuals can optimize their recovery journey and enhance their resilience in the face of challenges. Incorporating a variety of nutrient-dense foods into breakfast, lunch, and dinner meals ensures that your body receives the necessary fuel and building blocks for tissue repair, inflammation reduction, and optimal healing. With thoughtful meal planning, delicious recipes, and expert tips, individuals can nourish their bodies effectively and embark on a path toward sustained wellness and vitality.

CHAPTER 5
INCORPORATING ANTI-INFLAMMATORY FOODS

When undergoing osteotomy surgery, it's essential to pay close attention to your diet during the recovery period. One crucial aspect of this is incorporating anti-inflammatory foods into your meals. Inflammation is the body's natural response to injury or illness, but excessive inflammation can impede the healing process and exacerbate pain and discomfort. By understanding the role of inflammation and choosing foods rich in anti-inflammatory properties, you can support your body's healing process and promote overall wellness during recovery.

Knowledge of Inflammation and Its Effects

Inflammation is a complex biological response that occurs when the body's immune system recognizes an injury or infection. It's characterized by redness, swelling, heat, and pain, as the body works to repair damaged tissue and fight off pathogens. In acute situations, such as a sprained ankle or a cut, inflammation is a necessary and beneficial process that helps the body heal. However, chronic inflammation, which persists over an extended period, can lead to a range of health issues, including arthritis, cardiovascular disease, and autoimmune disorders.

For individuals undergoing osteotomy surgery, inflammation is a natural part of the healing process. The body responds to the trauma of surgery by initiating an inflammatory response to repair tissue damage and promote recovery. However, excessive inflammation can prolong recovery time, increase pain levels, and interfere with mobility and function. Therefore, managing inflammation through diet is crucial for optimizing the healing process and promoting long-term wellness.

Recipes Rich in Anti-Inflammatory Ingredients

Incorporating anti-inflammatory foods into your diet can help reduce inflammation, alleviate pain, and support overall health during the recovery period following osteotomy surgery. These foods are typically rich in antioxidants, vitamins, minerals, and phytochemicals that have been shown to modulate the body's inflammatory response. By including a variety of these ingredients in your meals, you can create delicious and nourishing dishes that promote healing and well-being.

One staple of an anti-inflammatory diet is fatty fish, such as salmon, mackerel, and sardines, which are rich in omega-3 fatty acids. Omega-3s have potent anti-inflammatory properties and have been shown to reduce levels of inflammatory markers in the body. Try incorporating grilled salmon into salads or making a comforting bowl of fish stew with tomatoes and leafy greens for a nutritious meal that supports healing.

Another anti-inflammatory powerhouse is turmeric, a spice commonly used in traditional Indian and Asian cuisine. Turmeric contains a compound called curcumin, which has been extensively studied for its anti-inflammatory and antioxidant effects. You can add turmeric to soups, stews, and curries for a vibrant color and flavor boost, or enjoy a soothing cup of turmeric tea to promote healing from within.

Leafy greens, such as kale, spinach, and Swiss chard, are also excellent additions to an anti-inflammatory diet. These greens are packed with vitamins, minerals, and phytonutrients that help combat inflammation and support overall health.

Try tossing together a colorful salad with mixed greens, cherry tomatoes, avocado, and a drizzle of olive oil and balsamic vinegar for a refreshing and nutrient-rich meal.

In addition to these specific ingredients, there are many other anti-inflammatory foods you can incorporate into your diet, including berries, nuts, seeds, and whole grains. Experiment with different recipes and meal combinations to discover what works best for you and your taste preferences.

By focusing on whole, unprocessed foods and avoiding excessive consumption of processed foods, sugar, and unhealthy fats, you can create a nourishing diet that supports your body's healing process and promotes long-term wellness after osteotomy surgery.

CHAPTER 6
HYDRATION AND FLUID INTAKE STRATEGIES

Ensuring adequate hydration is a crucial component of the recovery process following osteotomy surgery. Hydration plays a vital role in promoting tissue healing, maintaining electrolyte balance, supporting cellular function, and optimizing overall bodily functions. Therefore, implementing effective hydration and fluid intake strategies is essential for supporting the body's healing process and promoting optimal recovery outcomes.

Hydration Is Essential for Recovery:

Hydration is paramount during the recovery period after osteotomy surgery due to several reasons. Firstly, adequate hydration helps to maintain the body's fluid balance, which is essential for various physiological processes, including blood circulation, nutrient transport, and waste removal. Proper hydration also supports the function of vital organs, such as the kidneys, liver, and heart, facilitating the elimination of toxins and metabolic by-products from the body.

Moreover, hydration plays a crucial role in promoting tissue healing and repair. During the post-surgery period, the body requires an increased supply of nutrients and oxygen to support the regeneration of damaged tissues and promote wound healing. Optimal hydration ensures that these essential nutrients are effectively delivered to the injured tissues, facilitating the healing process and reducing the risk of complications such as infection or delayed wound healing.

Furthermore, maintaining adequate hydration levels can help alleviate common post-surgery symptoms such as fatigue, dizziness, and nausea. Dehydration can exacerbate these symptoms, leading to discomfort and delayed recovery. Therefore, staying well-hydrated is essential for managing post-surgery discomfort and promoting a smoother recovery experience.

To optimize hydration during the recovery period, it is important to adopt a multifaceted approach that includes both fluid intake and dietary strategies. Incorporating hydrating recipes and beverages into your post-surgery diet can help replenish lost fluids, electrolytes, and nutrients, supporting the body's healing process and promoting overall well-being.

Hydrating Recipes and Beverages:
When it comes to hydrating recipes and beverages for osteotomy surgery recovery, incorporating foods and drinks with high water content is key. These include:

1.   Fruit-infused water: Adding slices of fresh fruits such as lemon, cucumber, berries, or oranges

to plain water can enhance its flavor and increase its hydrating properties.

Fruit-infused water is refreshing and provides essential vitamins and minerals that support recovery.

2.   Herbal teas: Herbal teas, such as chamomile, peppermint, or ginger tea, are hydrating and can help alleviate post-surgery symptoms such as nausea and indigestion. They are also soothing and can promote relaxation, which is beneficial for recovery.

3.   Broth-based soups: Soups made with clear broths and plenty of vegetables are not only hydrating but also nutritious. Opt for broth-based soups with ingredients like carrots, celery, spinach, and lean protein sources such as chicken or tofu to provide essential nutrients for healing.

4.   Smoothies: Smoothies are an excellent way to increase fluid intake while also incorporating nutrient-dense ingredients into your diet. Blend

fruits, leafy greens, yogurt plant-based milk, and protein powder for a hydrating and nourishing beverage.

5.   Coconut water: Coconut water is a natural source of electrolytes, making it an ideal hydrating beverage for post-surgery recovery. It helps replenish lost electrolytes such as potassium and magnesium, which are essential for maintaining proper hydration and supporting muscle function.

In addition to incorporating hydrating recipes and beverages into your diet, it is essential to monitor your fluid intake throughout the day and adjust accordingly based on your individual needs and activity levels. Aim to drink at least 8-10 glasses of fluids per day, or more if you are experiencing increased sweating or fluid loss due to medications or other factors.

Furthermore, it is important to choose hydrating foods that are easy to digest and gentle on the stomach, especially during the initial stages of recovery when appetite and digestion may be compromised. Avoid foods and beverages that are high in sugar, caffeine, or alcohol, as they can have dehydrating effects and may interfere with the healing process.

By prioritizing hydration and incorporating hydrating recipes and beverages into your post-surgery diet, you can support the body's healing process, promote optimal recovery outcomes, and enhance overall well-being during the rehabilitation period following osteotomy surgery.

CHAPTER 7
SNACKS AND QUICK BITES FOR SUSTAINED ENERGY

In the journey of recovery following osteotomy surgery, the significance of nourishing your body with appropriate snacks and quick bites cannot be overstated. These interim meals play a pivotal role in sustaining energy levels, aiding the healing process, and ensuring optimal nutrition intake.

The period post-surgery demands a thoughtful approach towards dietary choices, focusing on foods that not only provide sustenance but also promote healing and recovery. This section delves into the realm of snacks and quick bites, offering insights into nutrient-dense options and convenient choices tailored to support your body's healing journey.

As you embark on the path of recovery, prioritizing nutrient-dense snack options is paramount for promoting healing and restoring vitality. Opting for snacks rich in essential vitamins, minerals, and macronutrients can facilitate tissue repair, bolster immune function, and alleviate postoperative discomfort. Incorporating a variety of nutrient-dense foods into your snack repertoire ensures a well-rounded nutritional intake, addressing the diverse needs of your healing body.

Fresh fruits emerge as a stellar choice for nutrient-dense snacking, delivering a plethora of vitamins, antioxidants, and fiber. Fruits such as berries, oranges, and kiwis not only offer a burst of flavor but also contribute to tissue regeneration and immune support. Pairing fruits with a source of protein, such as Greek yogurt or nuts, can enhance satiety and provide a sustained release of energy, making them an ideal snack option post-osteotomy surgery.

Vegetable-based snacks also stand out as nutritional powerhouses, brimming with essential nutrients vital for the healing process. Raw vegetable sticks paired with hummus or guacamole offer a crunchy, satisfying snack packed with vitamins, minerals, and phytonutrients. Additionally, incorporating roasted vegetables seasoned with herbs and spices provides a savory yet nutritious snack alternative, promoting healing and enhancing overall well-being.

Incorporating lean protein sources into your snack routine is instrumental in supporting muscle repair and promoting optimal recovery post-osteotomy surgery. Snack options such as hard-boiled eggs, grilled chicken skewers, or canned tuna offer a convenient and protein-rich way to nourish your body and facilitate healing. These protein-packed snacks not only help maintain muscle mass but also aid in wound healing and tissue regeneration, fostering a speedier recovery process.

Whole-grain snacks serve as a valuable source of complex carbohydrates, supplying sustained energy to fuel your body's healing endeavors.

Opt for whole-grain crackers topped with avocado or nut butter for a satisfying blend of carbohydrates, healthy fats, and protein. Alternatively, air-popped popcorn seasoned with herbs or nutritional yeast offers a wholesome, fiber-rich snack option that promotes satiety and supports digestive health.

Incorporating dairy or dairy alternatives into your snack repertoire provides a source of calcium and vitamin D crucial for bone health and healing post-osteotomy surgery. Choose low-fat cheese sticks, cottage cheese, or fortified plant-based yogurt to meet your calcium needs and promote optimal bone regeneration. Pairing dairy-based snacks with fruit or whole-grain crackers creates a balanced snack option that supports both healing and overall nutritional well-being.

Amid recovery, convenience plays a pivotal role in ensuring consistent nutritional intake throughout the day. Portable snacks offer a practical solution for nourishing your body on the go, enabling you to sustain energy levels and support healing even amidst a busy schedule. When selecting portable snack options post-osteotomy surgery, prioritizing convenience without compromising on nutritional quality is key to facilitating a seamless recovery journey.

Trail mix emerges as a convenient and versatile snack option, combining a variety of nuts, seeds, and dried fruits to deliver a nutrient-rich energy boost. Customize your trail mix with your preferred nuts and dried fruits, incorporating options such as almonds, walnuts, pumpkin seeds, and dried cranberries for a balanced blend of protein, healthy fats, and carbohydrates. Pre-portioned into individual servings, trail mix offers a convenient snack solution that can be easily packed and enjoyed on the go, supporting sustained energy and optimal nutrition throughout the day.

Protein bars present another portable snack option ideal for post-osteotomy surgery recovery, providing a convenient source of protein, carbohydrates, and essential nutrients in a compact form. Choose protein bars made with wholesome ingredients and minimal added sugars to support your body's healing process and promote long-term wellness. Look for options containing at least 10 grams of protein per serving, with a balanced macronutrient profile to sustain energy levels and promote muscle repair and recovery.

Pre-cut fruit and vegetable packs offer a convenient and hassle-free snack solution, delivering essential nutrients and hydration to support your body's healing journey. Opt for pre-packaged assortments of fresh fruit and vegetable slices, such as carrot sticks, cucumber rounds, and apple wedges, for a quick and nutritious snack option on the go.

 Pair with individual servings of hummus or Greek yogurt dip for added flavor and satiety, creating a well-rounded snack that nourishes your body and supports optimal recovery post-osteotomy surgery.

Individual servings of Greek yogurt or cottage cheese provide a convenient and protein-rich snack option that can be enjoyed anytime, anywhere.

Choose single-serving containers of Greek yogurt or cottage cheese for portion control and ease of transport, ensuring a steady supply of protein and calcium to support muscle repair and bone health post-osteotomy surgery. Enhance the flavor and nutritional value of your yogurt or cottage cheese with toppings such as fresh fruit, nuts, seeds, or a drizzle of honey for a satisfying and nourishing snack experience.

Portable smoothies offer a convenient and refreshing way to nourish your body with essential nutrients and hydration, supporting optimal recovery post-osteotomy surgery.

Blend your favorite fruits, leafy greens, protein powder, and liquid bases such as water, almond milk, or coconut water to create a nutrient-rich smoothie that fuels your body and promotes healing. Pour your smoothie into a portable insulated cup or bottle for on-the-go convenience, ensuring you have access to a nourishing snack wherever your recovery journey takes you.

CHAPTER 8
MANAGING DIGESTIVE HEALTH

Digestive health plays a crucial role in post-operative recovery, particularly following osteotomy surgery. The body's ability to efficiently process nutrients and eliminate waste is essential for healing and overall well-being. Therefore, implementing strategies to support digestive health becomes paramount during this recovery period. This section will delve into the importance of dietary fiber and gut-friendly recipes in promoting optimal digestive function post-osteotomy surgery.

Dietary Fiber for Digestive Support

Dietary fiber is a key component of a healthy diet, known for its ability to promote digestive health. Following osteotomy surgery, incorporating adequate amounts of fiber into the diet becomes even more crucial.

Fiber aids in maintaining regular bowel movements, preventing constipation, and promoting overall gastrointestinal function. Furthermore, fiber-rich foods can help reduce the risk of complications such as haemorrhoids, which may arise during the recovery period.

Fruits and vegetables are excellent sources of dietary fiber and should form a significant portion of the post-operative diet. Incorporating a variety of colorful fruits and vegetables ensures a diverse intake of essential vitamins, minerals, and antioxidants, in addition to fiber. Whole grains such as oats, quinoa, and brown rice are also rich in fiber and can be included in meals to support digestive health. Additionally, legumes like beans, lentils, and chickpeas provide a substantial amount of fiber and protein, further enhancing the nutritional value of post-operative meals.

It is essential to gradually increase fiber intake and stay hydrated to prevent any discomfort or digestive issues, especially during the initial stages of recovery. However, it's advisable to consult with a healthcare professional or a registered dietitian to determine the appropriate amount of fiber based on individual needs and tolerances. Overconsumption of fiber, particularly in the immediate postoperative period, may exacerbate gastrointestinal symptoms and should be avoided.

Gut-Friendly Recipes

Incorporating gut-friendly recipes into the post-osteotomy surgery recovery diet can significantly aid in digestive health and overall well-being. These recipes focus on incorporating nutrient-dense ingredients that are gentle on the digestive system while providing essential nutrients for healing and recovery. Here are some examples of gut-friendly recipes suitable for individuals recovering from osteotomy surgery:

1.   Creamy Vegetable Soup: This soothing soup combines a variety of vegetables such as carrots, celery, and zucchini, cooked until tender and blended to a creamy consistency. Adding a dash of turmeric and ginger not only enhances flavor but also provides anti-inflammatory properties, which can be beneficial during the healing process. Serve with a side of whole-grain bread or crackers for added fiber.

2.   Gentle Green Smoothie: A green smoothie packed with leafy greens like spinach or kale, along with ripe bananas, avocado, and a splash of coconut water or almond milk, is an excellent way to boost nutrient intake while being gentle on the digestive system. The fiber from the greens and fruits, combined with the healthy fats from avocado, provides a nourishing blend ideal for post-operative recovery.

3.   Mashed Sweet Potatoes: Mashed sweet potatoes are not only delicious but also easy to

digest, making them an ideal side dish for post-osteotomy surgery meals. Simply boil or roast sweet potatoes until soft, then mash with a bit of olive oil or coconut milk for creaminess. Season with a sprinkle of cinnamon or nutmeg for added flavor.

4.   Baked Salmon with Quinoa Salad: Salmon is rich in omega-3 fatty acids, which have anti-inflammatory properties and are beneficial for healing. Pairing baked salmon with a refreshing quinoa salad made with cucumber, cherry tomatoes, and fresh herbs creates a balanced and nutritious meal that supports digestive health. Drizzle with a light vinaigrette made with olive oil and lemon juice for added flavor.

5.   Chia Seed Pudding: Chia seeds are an excellent source of fiber and omega-3 fatty acids, making them a perfect ingredient for gut-friendly desserts. Combine chia seeds with almond milk or

coconut milk and a touch of sweeteners such as honey or maple syrup.

Allow the mixture to sit in the refrigerator until it thickens into a pudding-like consistency. Serve topped with fresh berries for added antioxidants and fiber.

These gut-friendly recipes are just a few examples of the many nutritious and delicious options available for individuals recovering from osteotomy surgery. By focusing on incorporating fiber-rich foods and gentle, easy-to-digest ingredients into meals, it is possible to support digestive health and promote optimal recovery. Experimenting with different recipes and consulting with a healthcare professional or registered dietitian can help tailor a post-operative diet plan to individual needs and preferences, ensuring long-term wellness and vitality.

CHAPTER 9
ADAPTATIONS FOR DIETARY RESTRICTIONS

In the realm of osteotomy surgery recovery, dietary adjustments play a pivotal role in facilitating healing, managing discomfort, and promoting overall wellness. While the focus remains on nourishing the body with essential nutrients, individuals may encounter dietary restrictions due to various reasons such as allergies, intolerances, or personal dietary choices. Understanding how to adapt to these restrictions ensures that individuals can still maintain a balanced diet conducive to recovery. Two common dietary restrictions include gluten-free and dairy-free diets, with vegan alternatives also gaining popularity for ethical and health reasons.

For individuals adhering to a gluten-free diet post-osteotomy surgery, navigating food choices can be challenging yet crucial for optimal recovery.

Gluten is a protein found in wheat, barley, rye, and their derivatives, which can trigger adverse reactions in those with celiac disease or gluten sensitivity. When planning a gluten-free recovery diet, it's essential to focus on naturally gluten-free whole foods such as fruits, vegetables, lean proteins, and gluten-free grains like quinoa, rice, and gluten-free oats.

When crafting meal plans, incorporating gluten-free substitutes for common staples like bread, pasta, and baked goods is essential. Fortunately, there is a wide array of gluten-free alternatives available in the market, including almond flour, coconut flour, tapioca flour, and gluten-free baking mixes. These alternatives not only provide texture and flavor but also ensure that individuals can enjoy familiar foods without compromising their dietary restrictions.

Moreover, paying attention to food labels and avoiding cross-contamination is imperative to maintain a strict gluten-free diet.

Reading ingredient lists thoroughly and opting for certified gluten-free products can help minimize the risk of inadvertently consuming gluten. Additionally, practicing safe food preparation techniques, such as using separate cooking utensils and kitchen equipment, can prevent cross-contact with gluten-containing ingredients.

Incorporating nutrient-dense foods rich in vitamins, minerals, and antioxidants is also essential for supporting the healing process and bolstering immune function. Foods like leafy greens, nuts, seeds, legumes, and gluten-free whole grains provide vital nutrients that aid in tissue repair and inflammation reduction, promoting faster recovery post-osteotomy surgery.

For individuals following dairy-free or vegan diets, adapting their nutrition during osteotomy surgery recovery requires careful consideration to ensure adequate nutrient intake without compromising on taste or variety. Dairy products are a common source of calcium and vitamin D, which are essential for bone health, making it crucial to find suitable alternatives that provide similar nutritional benefits.

Fortunately, numerous dairy-free alternatives are available, including plant-based milk alternatives such as almond milk, soy milk, coconut milk, and oat milk. These alternatives are fortified with calcium, vitamin D, and other nutrients to mimic the nutritional profile of dairy milk. Incorporating these alternatives into meals, such as using them in cereal, smoothies, or coffee, ensures individuals meet their calcium and vitamin D requirements without consuming dairy.

Moreover, replacing dairy-based cheeses and yogurts with plant-based alternatives made from nuts, seeds, or soy can provide similar flavor and texture while avoiding dairy-related discomfort or allergies. Additionally, incorporating sources of calcium-rich foods such as leafy greens, tofu, almonds, and fortified plant-based products into meals and snacks can further support bone health during the recovery process.

For individuals adhering to a vegan diet, ensuring adequate protein intake is essential for supporting muscle repair and overall recovery post-osteotomy surgery. Plant-based protein sources such as beans, lentils, chickpeas, quinoa, tofu, tempeh, and seitan can be incorporated into meals to meet protein requirements. Pairing these protein sources with whole grains, nuts, seeds, and vegetables not only enhances nutritional quality but also provides a well-rounded and satisfying dining experience.

adapting to dietary restrictions such as gluten-free, dairy-free, or vegan diets during osteotomy surgery recovery requires careful planning and consideration. By incorporating suitable alternatives, reading food labels, and focusing on nutrient-dense whole foods, individuals can ensure they maintain a balanced and nourishing diet conducive to optimal healing and long-term wellness. Consulting with a registered dietitian or healthcare professional can provide personalized guidance and support in navigating dietary restrictions and promoting recovery post-osteotomy surgery.

CHAPTER 10
MEAL PLANNING AND BATCH COOKING

Meal planning and batch cooking play integral roles in the recovery process after osteotomy surgery. This comprehensive guide aims to provide insights into these strategies to help individuals nourish their bodies effectively during the healing period. Following a well-thought-out meal plan and incorporating batch cooking into one's routine can significantly streamline the process of preparing nutritious meals while ensuring a balanced diet to support recovery.

Strategies for Efficient Meal Preparation

Efficient meal preparation begins with thoughtful planning and organization. When recovering from osteotomy surgery, it's essential to prioritize nutrient-dense foods that promote healing and support overall well-being.

One effective strategy is to plan meals, considering dietary restrictions, nutritional needs, and personal preferences.

This involves creating a weekly or monthly meal plan that includes a variety of foods rich in essential nutrients such as protein, vitamins, and minerals.

Another important aspect of efficient meal preparation is meal prepping. This involves prepping ingredients and meals ahead of time, making it easier to assemble and cook meals throughout the week. For example, chopping vegetables, marinating proteins, and cooking grains in advance can significantly reduce cooking time on busy days. Investing in quality food storage containers can also help prolong the freshness of prepped ingredients and meals.

Incorporating versatile ingredients into meal planning is another smart strategy. Opting for ingredients that can be used in multiple dishes can save time and minimize waste. For instance, roasted vegetables can be added to salads, grain bowls, or wraps, offering flexibility in meal options without requiring extensive cooking each time.

Furthermore, leveraging kitchen tools and appliances can streamline the cooking process. Using a slow cooker, Instant Pot, or air fryer can simplify meal preparation while enhancing flavor and texture. These appliances allow for hands-off cooking, freeing up time for other tasks while ensuring delicious and nutritious meals.

Lastly, staying organized and maintaining a well-stocked pantry and refrigerator is key to efficient meal preparation. Keeping staple ingredients such as grains, legumes, canned goods, and spices on hand ensures that you always have the foundation for nutritious meals. Regularly reviewing your pantry and making a shopping list based on your meal plan can help prevent last-minute trips to the grocery store and ensure that you have everything you need to stay on track with your recovery diet.

Batch Cooking Tips for Easy Meals

Batch cooking is a valuable technique for simplifying meal preparation and ensuring a steady supply of nourishing meals during the recovery period. By preparing large quantities of food in advance and portioning them out for future meals, individuals can save time and effort while still enjoying homemade meals packed with nutrients.

One of the key benefits of batch cooking is its ability to save time throughout the week. By dedicating a few hours to cooking in bulk, individuals can prepare several meals at once, eliminating the need for daily cooking sessions. This is particularly beneficial for those recovering from osteotomy surgery, as it reduces the physical strain of standing and cooking for extended periods.

When batch cooking, it's essential to focus on recipes that are suitable for freezing and reheating without compromising taste or texture. Casseroles, soups, stews, and sauces are excellent options for batch cooking, as they tend to improve in flavor over time and can be easily portioned out and stored for later use. Additionally, incorporating a variety of proteins, vegetables, and grains into batch-cooked meals ensures a well-rounded and nutritious diet.

Proper storage is critical when batch cooking to maintain the quality and safety of the prepared meals. Investing in high-quality food storage containers that are freezer-friendly and microwave-safe is essential for preserving the freshness of batch-cooked meals. Labeling containers with the date and contents can help keep track of what's in the freezer and ensure that meals are consumed within a reasonable timeframe.

Incorporating batch cooking into a weekly meal routine requires careful planning and organization. Setting aside dedicated time for batch cooking, such as on weekends or days off, allows individuals to focus on preparing meals without distractions. Creating a meal plan and shopping list beforehand ensures that you have all the necessary ingredients on hand, minimizing the risk of running out of key components midway through cooking.

Batch cooking also offers the opportunity to experiment with new recipes and flavor combinations. By preparing larger quantities of food, individuals can afford to be more adventurous in their cooking endeavors, trying out different spices, herbs, and ingredients to enhance the taste and nutritional value of their meals.

This can help prevent boredom with the recovery diet and keep mealtimes exciting and enjoyable.

meal planning and batch cooking are essential strategies for nourishing the body during the recovery period after osteotomy surgery.

By incorporating these techniques into one's routine, individuals can simplify meal preparation, save time and effort, and ensure a steady supply of nutritious meals to support healing and overall well-being.

With careful planning, organization, and creativity, mealtime can be a pleasurable and nourishing experience, contributing to long-term health and wellness.

CHAPTER 11
FAMILY-FRIENDLY RECIPES FOR EVERYONE

Osteotomy surgery, a procedure aimed at correcting deformities or realigning bones, requires careful attention not only during the operation and immediate post-operative phase but also throughout the recovery period. One crucial aspect of recovery is maintaining a balanced and nourishing diet, which aids in healing, supports overall health, and facilitates the body's ability to regain strength. In the context of osteotomy surgery recovery, the significance of a well-rounded diet cannot be overstated. It plays a pivotal role in promoting optimal recovery, managing inflammation, and ensuring the body receives essential nutrients vital for tissue repair and overall wellness.

Children undergoing osteotomy surgery or those whose family members are recovering from such procedures require special attention when it comes to nutrition. Ensuring they receive adequate nourishment is crucial for their growth, development, and recovery. However, children can often be picky eaters, making it challenging for caregivers to provide them with nutritious meals that they'll enjoy. Kid-friendly meals tailored to their tastes and preferences can make the recovery period more manageable and enjoyable for both children and their caregivers. These meals should incorporate a balance of nutrients essential for healing and growth while appealing to children's palates.

When preparing kid-friendly meals for those recovering from osteotomy surgery, it's essential to focus on incorporating foods rich in protein, vitamins, and minerals necessary for tissue repair and overall health.

Lean proteins such as chicken, turkey, fish, and tofu can provide the building blocks needed for muscle and tissue repair. Additionally, including a variety of colorful fruits and vegetables ensures a good intake of essential vitamins, antioxidants, and fiber, supporting the body's healing process and boosting the immune system.

Moreover, incorporating whole grains such as brown rice, quinoa, and whole wheat bread provides sustained energy levels and essential nutrients like B vitamins and fiber. For children who may have specific dietary restrictions or preferences, creativity in meal preparation can be key. Transforming nutritious ingredients into fun and visually appealing dishes can make mealtime more enjoyable for children and encourage them to eat a balanced diet.

Support from loved ones plays a significant role in the recovery journey of individuals undergoing osteotomy surgery.

Whether it's preparing meals, providing emotional support, or assisting with daily tasks, the presence of a supportive network can greatly enhance the recovery process. In the context of nutrition, loved ones can contribute by preparing nourishing meals that cater to the specific dietary needs of the recovering individual.

Recipes designed for sharing with loved ones should focus on simplicity, versatility, and nutrient density. These meals should be easy to prepare, transport, and reheat, allowing caregivers to provide support without added stress. Additionally, they should be adaptable to accommodate any dietary restrictions or preferences of the recovering individual, ensuring they receive meals that align with their nutritional needs.

One approach to creating recipes for sharing is to focus on batch cooking or meal prepping. By preparing large quantities of nutritious meals in advance, caregivers can ensure that the recovering individual has access to wholesome food throughout their recovery period. This approach not only saves time and effort but also allows for greater variety in meals, preventing monotony and enhancing the overall dining experience.

When selecting recipes for sharing with loved ones, it's essential to prioritize ingredients known for their healing properties and nutritional benefits. Incorporating foods rich in anti-inflammatory compounds, such as omega-3 fatty acids found in fatty fish, nuts, and seeds, can help reduce inflammation and promote faster recovery. Additionally, including ingredients high in antioxidants, such as berries, leafy greens, and cruciferous vegetables, supports cellular repair and boosts immune function.

providing nourishing meals during the recovery period following osteotomy surgery is essential for promoting healing, supporting overall health, and enhancing the well-being of the individual undergoing surgery.

By focusing on kid-friendly meals tailored to children's tastes and preferences and creating recipes for sharing with loved ones that prioritize simplicity, versatility, and nutrient density, caregivers can play a vital role in facilitating the recovery process and ensuring the best possible outcomes for their loved ones.

CONCLUSION

navigating osteotomy surgery and the subsequent recovery period can be a challenging journey, but with the right tools and knowledge, it can also be a time of profound healing and transformation.

This comprehensive guide has provided a roadmap for nourishing your body throughout this process, offering not only healing recipes and meal plans but also expert tips for long-term wellness.

Throughout the chapters, we've delved into the importance of understanding osteotomy surgery and its recovery process, emphasizing the crucial role that nutrition plays in facilitating healing. From stocking your kitchen with essential ingredients to incorporating key nutrients like protein, carbohydrates, and healthy fats into your meals, each aspect has been carefully considered to support your body's needs during this critical time.

We've explored strategies for managing inflammation, staying hydrated, and maintaining digestive health, recognizing the interconnectedness of these factors in promoting overall well-being. Moreover, we've addressed common dietary restrictions, ensuring that individuals with gluten-free, dairy-free, or vegan lifestyles can still find nourishing options tailored to their needs.

Practical advice on meal planning, batch cooking, and creating family-friendly recipes has been provided to make the process more manageable and enjoyable for everyone involved.

By implementing these strategies, you can not only support your recovery but also foster a sense of togetherness and support within your household.

As you embark on this journey toward healing and long-term wellness, remember that nourishing your body is not just about physical sustenance but also about caring for your mental and emotional well-being. Be patient with yourself, listen to your body's needs, and lean on your support network for guidance and encouragement. With dedication and perseverance, you can emerge from this experience stronger, healthier, and more resilient than ever before.